The Healing Oils of Ancient Scripture

Rebecca Park Totilo

The Healing Oils of Ancient Scripture

Scripture references are taken from the King James Version of the Bible.

Disclaimer Notice: The information contained in this book is intended for educational purposes only and is not meant to substitute for medical care or prescribe treatment for any specific health condition. Please see a qualified health care provider for medical treatment. We assume no responsibility or liability for any person or group for any loss, damage or injury resulting from the use or misuse of any information in this book. No express or implied guarantee is given regarding the effects of using any of the products described herein.

ISBN 978-0-9749115-6-4

Table of Contents

Introduction

Twelve of the most highly-praised fragrances are presented in Holy Scripture. These include: Spikenard, Galbanum, Frankincense, Myrrh, Cypress, Cedarwood, Aloes/Sandalwood, Rose of Sharon, Cassia/Cinnamon, Hyssop, Onycha, and Myrtle. While some perfumers have used these names to label their own formulas, only the attributes of the biblical oils that are pure, therapeutic grade essential oils from all over the world will be discussed.

Aromatic plants, herbs and oils have been used for incense, perfume, culinary and medicinal purposes for thousands of years by many cultures. Since ancient times, spices and oils have been an integral part of the Hebraic culture. The Bible mentions over 33 species of fragrant plants with over 1,035 references to essential oils and/or plants in the Old and New Testaments.

People of the Holy Land understood the use of essential oils in maintaining wellness and physical healing, as well as the oils' ability to enhance their spiritual state in worship, prayer and confession, and for cleansing and purification from sin. During biblical times, essential oils were inhaled, applied to the body, and taken internally in which the benefits extended to every aspect of their being.

Most Jewish households employed essential oils for medicinal and household purposes. One example in Scripture is the parable Yeshua told of the Good Samaritan who was carrying oil and wine and helped the injured man that had been robbed and left for dead.

Essential oils can be emotionally, spiritually, mentally, and physically healing and transform diseased tissue into thriving, healthy cells. Unfortunately, people today have become dependent upon and rely heavily upon medicine. In many cases it helps, but for most their faith has been placed in doctors instead of God. In an article entitled "Death by Medicine," published by Nutrition Institute of America, four doctors stated that almost 800,000 deaths occur each year due to drug interaction.[1]

The Scriptures show that God gave natural herbs, including their extracts, for medicines. Ezekiel 47:12 reads:

> "And by the river upon the bank thereof, on this side and on that side, shall grow all trees for meat, whose leaf shall not fade, neither shall the fruit thereof be consumed: it shall bring forth new fruit according to his months, because their waters they issued out of the sanctuary: and the fruit thereof shall be for meat, and the leaf thereof for medicine."

And in Revelation 22:2, it reads:

---

[1] Null, Gary, MD, Martin Feldman, MD, Deborah Rasio, MD, and Dorothy Smith, Ph.D. "Death by Medicine." Nutrition Institute of America. October 2003.

"In the midst of the street of it, and on either side of the river, *was there* the tree of life, which bare twelve *manner of* fruits, *and* yielded her fruit every month: and the leaves of the tree *were* for the healing of the nations."

Fragrances of the Bible come from plant essences or the life-blood of the plant. The two types of oils plants make are *essential* and *fatty*. Most seeds contain both types of oils. Essential oils circulate within a plant to carry out its function as a living creation, while the fatty oils remain in the seed where they serve as food for the young plant, as God intended. Fragrant essential oils are also how they communicate to the rest of the animal kingdom and mankind. Plants use their odors to attract insects and animals to pollinate, with fragrances disappearing within 30 minutes of being pollinated.

For perfumers, this is important when extracting oils from flowers. When extracting, it is crucial to do it at the right time before the desired aromatic essential oil has been chemically altered.

While fatty vegetable oil from the seed serves as nourishment for the small plant, it cannot enter the blood stream nor cross the blood-brain barrier. The molecules of fatty oils are too large to evaporate and circulate through the tissues of the body. Their uses in aromatherapy are for providing a neutral lipid base in which essential oils can be blended and/or diluted for massage use when an essential oil is too strong.[2]

---

[2] Stewart, David, Ph.D., D.N.M. The Chemistry of Essential Oils Made Simple: God's love manifest in molecules. Care Publications. 2005. Page 59.

Essentials oils were God's original medicine, created on the third day. When God created these plants, His word went forth in power creating life and continues to create life in the life-blood of the plant, which is the oil. Genesis 1:12-13 says:

> "And the earth brought forth grass, *and* herb yielding seed after his kind, and the tree yielding fruit, whose seed *was* in itself, after his kind: and God saw that *it was* good. And the evening and the morning were the third day."

Myrrh

In Esther 2:12 the Bible describes Esther's preparations for becoming queen which involved six months with the oil of Myrrh, a spice commonly used for preparing bodies for burial.

A similar custom is described in the Song of Solomon revealing another bridal tradition concerning the use of Myrrh. In the Song of Solomon 1:13, the bride responds to the king and says, "A bundle of myrrh *is* my wellbeloved unto me; he shall lie all night betwixt my breasts." This reflects a popular custom of laying a bundle of Myrrh on one's chest while sleeping as a beauty treatment in preparation for a wedding. Both of these examples from the Word teach believers that the first step to becoming the Bride of Messiah is to spiritually put the flesh to death.

Most believers know from experience the works of the flesh are the first issues God deals with when they come to know Yeshua as their Savior. The Scriptures list these works in Galatians 5:19-21:

"Now the works of the flesh are manifest, which are *these*; Adultery, fornication, uncleanness, lasciviousness, idolatry, witchcraft, hatred, variance, emulations, wrath, strife, seditions, heresies, envyings, murders, drunkenness, revellings, and such like: of which I tell you before, as I have also told *you* in time past, that they which do such things shall not inherit the kingdom of God."

Esther didn't do it alone, as Scripture shows. She had the king's eunuch Hegai to guide her in how to prepare. Believers also have a guide—the Holy Spirit—showing them all things in how to ready themselves for His return.

In the same way Esther prepared, the Spirit provides His betrothed ones with oil of Myrrh, which represents the fellowship of His sufferings, being conformed to His death.

Philippians 3:10-11 reads, "That I may know him, and the power of his resurrection, and the fellowship of his sufferings, being made conformable unto his death; if by any means I might attain unto the resurrection of the dead."

Because of what Yeshua did, the Lord's Bride can share in His victory over sin, the world, and the flesh!

Tears of Myrrh

During the Messiah's final agonizing hours in the Garden of Gethsemane, the weight of the world's sins crushed the Savior like a wine press, causing Him to sweat great tears of blood.

His bitter sufferings can be compared to Myrrh, a highly-prized spice used for perfumes and incense, extracted by piercing the tree's heartwood and allowing the gum to trickle out and harden into bitter, aromatic red droplets called "tears."

The Hebrew word for Myrrh is *mowr*, which means "distilled" and comes from the root word *marar*, which means "bitterness."

After the Savior's crucifixion, His body was prepared with Myrrh. As a member of Yeshua's body, believers are to be made ready with the burial of their sins at the cross. They must die to the old life, as death is the first step in preparation for those who will become the Bride of the Messiah.

Yeshua told His disciples in Matthew 16:24b-25, "If any *man* will come after me, let him deny himself, and take up his cross, and follow me. For whosoever will save his life shall lose it: and whosoever will lose his life for my sake shall find it."

As joint heirs with the Messiah, His Bride is to share in His affliction according to 2 Corinthians 1:5, so that she can be triumphant through the bitterness of suffering. Believers are told to rejoice in this. Colossians 1:24 says, "Who now rejoice in my sufferings for you, and fill up that which is behind of the afflictions of Christ in my flesh for his body's sake."

Myrrh is a fixing or servant oil which is used by apothecaries to enhance the fragrance of the other oils and make them last longer. Isn't that just like the Messiah? He is a servant and desires to lift up His Bride and enhance her with beautiful things.

The First and the Last

Rich with symbolism, Myrrh is mentioned 156 times in the Bible. It is the first oil mentioned in the Bible in Genesis 37:25, when Joseph's jealous brothers sold him into slavery to a caravan of Ishmaelites (incense traders) who were on their way to Egypt, carrying "balm and myrrh." Years later during the famine, Joseph's brothers came to Egypt to buy food, encountering Joseph as an Egyptian prince.

Interestingly, Jacob their father (now called Israel) told his sons to take gifts for the prince. The Scripture says they brought Joseph balm and Myrrh (Genesis 43:11)—the same two oils that accompanied Joseph into slavery.

Not only is Myrrh the first oil mentioned in the Bible, it is the last one mentioned in Revelation 18:13: "And cinnamon, and odours, and ointments ("myrrh" in the Greek), and frankincense, and wine, and oil, and fine flour, and wheat, and beasts, and sheep, and horses, and chariots, and slaves, and souls of men."

Myrrh was one of the first gum resins/oils given as a gift to Yeshua as a young child by the Magi in Matthew 2:11. It was also the last oil offered to Yeshua at Golgotha when He was crucified. In Mark 15:23, it says, "And they gave him to drink wine mingled with myrrh: but he received *it* not."

Therapeutic/Medicinal Uses

Myrrh was known to act as a pain-reliever, which is why the Romans mixed it to the sour wine and offered it to Yeshua on the cross.[3]

Recent studies and medicinal research has discovered that Myrrh is anti-infectious, antiviral, anti-parasitic, hormone-like, anti-inflammatory, and anti-hyperthyroid. It soothes skin conditions and supports the immunity system.[4,5]

Dr. Mohamed Rafi at Rutgers University discovered Myrrh to be anti-cancer and effective for prevention and treatment of breast and prostrate cancer, according to the Journal of Natural Products.[6]

Other uses include treating bronchitis, diarrhea, dysentery, hyperthyroidism, stretch marks and skin conditions, eczema, gingivitis, gum infections, asthma, athlete's foot, thrush and vaginal thrush, ulcers, and viral hepatitis.[7,8]

---

[3] Dolara, P. "Analgesic Effects of Myrrh." Nature. 4 January 1996.
[4] Essential Oils Desk Reference. Essential Science Publishing.
[5] Farres-Hall, Gill. The Aromatherapy Bible. Sterling Publishing. Page 314.
[6] Rutgers University professor and co-researcher, Mohamed M. Rafi, Ph.D., identified an anti-cancer compound in Myrrh and believed it could be developed into a potent drug for the prevention and treatment of breast and prostrate cancer. This information was published in the Journal of Natural Products on November 26, 2001.
[7] Essential Oils Desk Reference. Essential Science Publishing.
[8] Sibley, Veronica. Aromatherapy Solutions: Essential oils to lift the mind, body, and spirit.

"Nature" magazine reported in an article entitled "Analgesic Effects of Myrrh," that Myrrh promotes a feeling of security.[9] Many find just inhaling the fragrance lifts the spirit.

---

[9] Dolara, P. "Analgesic Effects of Myrrh." <u>Nature</u>. 4 January 1996.

Spice Chest: How Essential Oils Work

Clinical research has discovered that essentials oils have the highest frequency of any natural substance. Electrical properties and charges of essential oils carry electrons or negative ions, which are healing and healthful.[10]

A healthy human body ranges from 62 to 68 MHz. The air breathed, food eaten, and other factors cause frequency levels to drop. Examples of the Taino Technology study reveal:

At 58 MHz cold and flu symptoms may appear.
At 55 MHz diseases like Candida and arthritis may take hold.
At 42 MHz cancer may set in.
At 25 MHz death begins.[11]

The essence or life-blood of the plant carries a live frequency—ranging from 52 MHz to 320 MHz.

Using therapeutic grade essential oils on a daily basis keeps body frequencies at a healthy level, prevents disease, and even reverses damage.

---

[10] Researchers used a biofrequency monitor from Taino Technology to measure the biofrequency of essential oils.
[11] Ibid.

Research has shown that the number one cause for depression is the loss of oxygen around the pineal and pituitary glands. They have also discovered that with careful application of these oils to the soles of the feet, it enables the oil to reach every cell in the body within 20 minutes.[12] This may be why people in biblical times lived so long.

Principal essential oils contain various constituents, including these three compounds: phenylpropanoids, sesquiterpenes, and monoterpenes.[13] These three constituents are unique to essential oils and are produced naturally by the plant with the intelligence and capacity to do the following:

Phenylpropanoids - cleanse the receptor sites.
Sesquiterpenes - erase the incorrect information in the DNA or cellular memory.
Monoterpenes - reprogram the cellular intelligence back to God's original plan with correct information.

Sesquiterpenes carry oxygen to the brain and stimulate the pineal and pituitary glands. Three of the four oils in the world with the highest known concentration of sesquiterpenes are biblical oils: Cedarwood, Sandalwood, and Spikenard.

---

[12] Vabener, Dr. Seminar Course. University of Izmir in Turkey. 1996.
[13] Stewart, David, Ph.D., D.N.M. Healing Oils of the Bible. Care Publications. 2003. Page 30-31.

Rose of Sharon

In ancient times, the Cistus Ladanifer, also known as the "rock rose," was believed to be the Rose of Sharon. As goats and sheep roamed through the brush, this flower became entangled in their coats. While caring for their sheep, the shepherds would collect it from their wool and rub the resin on their cuts and wounds to soothe them.

This multi-petal flower is found in the fertile plain called Sharon between Jaffa and Mount Carmel in Israel. It has a honey scent from an aromatic gum that exudes from the plant.

The Hebrew word *sharon* means "meadow-saffron, crocus, and rose (place of pasture)." It is a derivative for Sarai, which means "princess."

Think of how the thornless Rose of Sharon beautifully mirrors Yeshua's tender love, as spoken of in Song of Solomon 2:1: "I *am* the rose of Sharon, *and* the lily of the valleys." The Scriptures tell believers that they are the sheep of His pasture and feed among the lilies.

Therapeutic/Medicinal Uses

Rose of Sharon has been studied for its therapeutic effect on cell regeneration according to Dr. David Stewart, author of "Healing Oils of the Bible."[14]

Rose of Sharon has been used for bronchitis, respiratory infections, urinary tract infections, wounds, and wrinkles. It is also known to be anti-infectious, antiviral, and antibacterial. Rose of Sharon helps to reduce inflammation and acts as a powerful anti-hemorrhaging agent. The Essential Oils Desk Reference reports that it also helps strengthen the immune system.[15]

Rose of Sharon helps to quiet the nerves and elevate the emotions during prayer. Studies revealed that people taking antidepressant drugs found this oil to be mood-elevating by rubbing it on their bodies or just inhaling it.[16]

---

[14] Stewart, David, Ph.D., D.N.M. Healing Oils of the Bible. Care Publications. 2003. Page 218.
[15] Essential Oils Desk Reference. Essential Science Publishing.
[16] Higley, Alan and Conni. Reference Guide to Essential Oils. Abundant Health.

Spice Chest: The Sense of Smell

Smelling the fragrance of a rose can bring healing and elevate one's mood. Even when the scent is too faint to notice healing is taking place. The sense of smell facilitated through the olfactory nerve invites the fragrance into certain regions of the brain, enabling the body to process them naturally.

Just inhaling a fragrance will bring healing to the body because with pure therapeutic essential oils the molecules are small enough to bypass the blood-brain barrier and reach down at the cellular level to bring healing.[17] Regular inhalation of essential oils stimulates the limbic region of the brain and encourages the natural release of the human growth hormone (HGH).[18]

With 1,000 sensors in the nose, it can identify 10,000 scents.[19] And because the nose is wired differently that the other four senses, it carries molecules directly into the emotional center of

---

[17] Stewart, David, Ph.D., D.N.M. The Chemistry of Essential Oils Made Simple: God's love manifest in molecules. Care Publications. 2005.
[18] Ledoux, Dr. Joseph. New York Medical University.
[19] Cromie, William. "Researchers Sniff Out Secrets of Smell." Harvard University Gazette.

the brain where traumatic memories are stored. Essential oils are a vehicle by which repressed emotions can be released.[20]

The Hebrew word for "smell" is *reyach*, and this shares the same root word for "spirit," which is *ruach*. Yahweh was moved to compassion through the sense of smell as in the account of Noah's offering after the flood: "And Noah builded an altar unto the LORD... and offered burnt offerings... and the LORD smelled a sweet savour; and the LORD said in his heart, I will not again curse the ground any more for man's sake" (Genesis 8:20-21).

---

[20] Stewart, David, Ph.D., D.N.M. Healing Oils of the Bible. Care Publications. 2003. Page 32-33.

Cassia/Cinnamon

Cassia and Cinnamon are mentioned in Exodus 30:22-31 as part of the holy anointing oil. The Hebrew word for the spice *Cassia* is similar to the word meaning "to bow down or to pay homage." "Homage" in the Scriptures means "to honor another by bending low in deep respect." Yeshua's Bride is to be humble toward all people. She is to bow down in homage to God alone.

Cassia and Cinnamon are very similar in fragrance because they are actually of the same genus and the laurel family of plants. Cassia was considered inferior to other plants in the laurel family.[21]

Isn't that true of Yeshua's life? The leaders considered Him of little account because He came from Nazareth, but His Father glorified Him, as mentioned in John 8:54.

In the middle ages, the Arabs maintained monopoly of the spice trade by claiming Cinnamon was harvested from the nests of ferocious birds and had to be gathered under their attack.[22]

This prized spice was also used by a band of thieves who stole jewels off dead bodies during the Black Plague in Europe

---

[21] United States Department of Agriculture.
[22] Aromatherapy Solutions. Page 67.

without contracting the disease. When the King of England questioned them, he discovered that their secret was essential oils, which included Cinnamon.

Therapeutic/Medicinal Uses

Both Cassia and Cinnamon are extremely effective in fighting bacteria and viruses. Research has revealed that most viruses, fungi, and bacteria cannot sustain themselves in the presence of therapeutic grade essential oils and it was probably these oils that protected the Israelites from disease.[23]

Benefits of Cassia oil include offering support to the immunity system against colds and flu simply by inhaling them or rubbing them on the soles of the feet.

Cinnamon is being used to cure diabetes, high-blood sugar, and high blood pressure according to the U.S. Department of Agriculture.[24] It also calms spasms of the digestive tract, indigestion, diarrhea, colitis, vomiting, and nausea. Many have used Cinnamon for the treatment of depression and stress-related conditions.

These oils may also be used for dry, sensitive skin, but both should be diluted with a carrier oil such as olive oil.

---

[23] Stewart, David, Ph.D., D.N.M. The Chemistry of Essential Oils Made Simple: God's love manifest in molecules. Care Publications. 2005. Page 129.
[24] United States Department of Agriculture.

Spice Chest: The Scent of His Coming

When Yeshua returns, the world will smell His coming! His garments will be scented with these biblical fragrances. Psalm 45:7-8 says:

> "Thou lovest righteousness, and hatest wickedness: therefore God, thy God, hath anointed thee with the oil of gladness above thy fellows. All thy garments *smell* of myrrh, and aloes, *and* cassia, out of the ivory palaces, whereby they have made thee glad."

These fragrances burn as incense before the throne of Yah and Yeshua's fragrance fills the Temple. Revelation 8:3-4 says:

> "And another angel came and stood at the altar, having a golden censer; and there was given unto him much incense, that he should offer *it* with the prayers of all saints upon the golden altar which was before the throne. And the smoke of the incense, *which came* with the prayers of the saints, ascended up before God out of the angel's hand."

Cedarwood

Cedarwood has been used for over 5,000 years by the Egyptians and the Sumerians for ritual purposes. Other uses included embalming, a disinfectant, and other medicinal purposes.

Cedars of Lebanon is the highest in sesquiterpenes (98%) which oxygenates the brain and supports clear thinking. The Scriptures record that Solomon built the Temple and his palace out of the Cedars of Lebanon—which may be why Solomon was the wisest man to ever live.

Spiritually, Cedar is symbolic of strength and serves as a hedge of protection. In Song of Solomon 1:17, it speaks about the boards of Cedarwood: "The beams of our house *are* cedar, *and* our rafters of fir." A bride's trousseau or "cedar chest," which holds her treasures, protects her valuables from moths, silverfish, and other infestations. A believer's heart is where God's treasure is. Yeshua reminds believers to guard their hearts from the enemy, who wants to come in and steal their joy and peace.

For practical purposes, this oil serves well as an insect repellant. Its scent stays in the wood for a lifetime, even after the wood has been made into furniture—and it is this same fragrance which inhibits the growth of bacteria.

Therapeutic/Medicinal Uses

Cedarwood is effective against hair loss, tuberculosis, bronchitis, gonorrhea, urinary infections, acne, and psoriasis.[25] It also helps in reducing the hardening of the artery wall and stimulates the pineal gland to release natural melatonin for deep sleep.[26] Cedarwood clears the mind and eases ADD.[27]

The thumb and big toe are trigger points for clearing fears of the unknown and mental blocks against learning.[28] The big toe is also a point for clearing addictions and compulsive behavior. The scent of Cedarwood helps to clear buried emotions, including pride and conceit.

---

[25] Cooksley, Valerie Gennari, R.N. Aromatherapy.
[26] Taken from a study conducted by the America Academy of Reflexology, published in "Obstetrics and Gynecology," Volume 82, Number 6, December 1993.
[27] Ibid.
[28] Ibid.

Hyssop

King David wrote in Psalm 51:7, "Purge me with hyssop, and I shall be clean: wash me, and I shall be whiter than snow."

David prayed this prayer after Nathan the prophet came and confronted him about his sin of going in to Bathsheba, committing adultery and murder (2 Samuel 12:1-14).

As he began to meditate on the law, David felt great remorse and truly repented from his sin. He wanted to restore his relationship with God. His understanding of the healing properties of Hyssop as a purifier inspired him in his psalm of prayer to God.

The Hebrew word for "Hyssop" is *esob*, and means "holy herb." Hyssop is considered to be spiritually purifying and serves as an aid in cleansing oneself from sin, immorality, evil thoughts, or bad habits.

The method of using of Hyssop oil (inhaled or applied to the body) to purge oneself from iniquity has scientific basis.

Hyssop has constituents that can reprogram the DNA where sinful tendencies (negative emotions) are stored, thus releasing and cleansing the root cause of the action.[29]

Another reason for Jewish belief that Hyssop repels evil spirits is because of the passage in the book of Exodus, where Moses asked the elders of Israel to sacrifice a spotless lamb and to use a Hyssop branch to apply the blood of the lamb to the doorposts of their dwellings.

At the first Passover, the angel of death killed the firstborn son of every household except those whose doorway was marked with the lamb's blood using a Hyssop branch. Exodus 12:22 says, "And ye shall take a bunch of hyssop, and dip *it* in the blood that *is* in the bason, and strike the lintel and the two side posts with the blood that *is* in the bason." Striking the doorposts would have released the scent of the Hyssop and the oil.

Yeshua, who died in His Bride's place, became the Passover Lamb. In John 19:29, it reads, "Now there was set a vessel full of vinegar: and they filled a spunge with vinegar, and put *it* upon hyssop, and put *it* to his mouth."

They dipped the sponge in sour wine or vinegar and extended it to His mouth on a branch of Hyssop, because He is the door. This prophetic charade portrayed His blood as the only way

---

[29] Stewart, David, Ph.D., D.N.M. The Chemistry of Essential Oils Made Simple: God's love manifest in molecules. Care Publications. 2005. Page 304.

of salvation and the Hyssop—symbolic of the Holy Spirit—as the one who purifies and sanctifies the believer.

Therapeutic/Medicinal Uses

Valerie Cooksley, R.N., wrote in her book "Aromatherapy" the uses of Hyssop as anti-inflammatory, antioxidant, anti-parasitic, antiseptic, and antiviral.[30]

Hyssop is good for easing colds, coughs, and fever as a decongestant. It helps reduce fat in tissue, raises low blood pressure, opens the respiratory system, and strengthens and tones the nervous system. Hyssop serves as a sedative and is good for quieting anxiety and clearing the mind.[31]

---

[30] Cooksley, Valerie Gennari, R.N. Aromatherapy. Page 351.
[31] George Nemecz, Ph.D., assistant professor of biochemistry at the Campbell University School of Pharmacy.

Spice Chest: Anointing of the Feet

In biblical times, it was customary for visitors traveling long distances over dusty roads to be welcomed warmly with a foot-washing followed by anointing with oil as an expression of Jewish hospitality. This is mentioned in Genesis 18:4 and Genesis 24:32.

In the New Testament, Yeshua made mention of this custom when He was invited to a Pharisee's house for dinner and they did not extend this act of hospitality to Him.

In the gospel of Luke, Yeshua was anointed by an uninvited woman at this gathering where she washed His feet with her tears and then wiped them with her hair. In Luke 7:36-38, it says:

"And one of the Pharisees desired him that he would eat with him. And he went into the Pharisee's house, and sat down to meat. And, behold, a woman in the city, which was a sinner, when she knew that *Jesus* sat at meat in the Pharisee's house, brought an alabaster box of ointment, and stood at his feet behind *him* weeping, and begun to wash his feet with tears, and did wipe *them* with the hairs of her head, and kissed his feet, and anointed *them* with the ointment."

Spikenard

Spikenard comes from a very rare plant that is usually blended with olive oil for anointing acts of consecration, dedication, and worship. The Greek word for "Spikenard" means "genuine or pure."

There are three accounts in the Scriptures of Yeshua being anointed with Spikenard, found in Luke 7:36-38, Mark 14:3 and in John 12:1-3.[32]

Pure Spikenard is a very costly spice and the word "nard," used in the King James Version, is from the Hebrew word *nard* meaning "light." The Scriptures describe Yeshua in Mark 9:3, when He was transfigured and His whiteness was beyond any earthly whiteness.[33]

Those desiring to become the spotless Bride of Messiah must walk in purity and light, burying sins at the stake. With His life broken, He doesn't leave believers alone to "waste away." Instead, the oil, symbolic of the inner working of the *Ruach HaKodesh*, has been poured out, so believers can live a life that is rich with a sweet,

---

[32] "The Life of Jesus Christ" Collectors Edition, Disc 1. Courtesy of Diamond Entertainment, copyrighted.
[33] Totilo, Rebecca Park. The Hebrew Wedding Customs. 2005.

heavenly fragrance. Song of Solomon 1:12 says, "While the king *sitteth* at his table, my spikenard sendeth forth the smell thereof."

The King is sitting, symbolic of His finished work at the cross. He invites His Bride to come and join Him for a feast at His table. Here is a picture of the Bride and her fragrance is emanating out of her spirit in worship to the King's provision. It is a heavenly fragrance all should possess.

Solomon's prophecy was fulfilled a thousand years later in John 12:3, where the Bible tells how Spikenard was used to anoint Yeshua, the pure and spotless Lamb, just days before His death and burial: "Then took Mary a pound of ointment of spikenard, very costly, and anointed the feet of Jesus, and wiped his feet with her hair: and the house was filled with the odour of the ointment."

Some of the disciples were very indignant with the "waste" of costly oil, as it may have cost this woman as much as a whole year's wages. But Yeshua rebuked them and said she had done a good work, preparing Him for His death. And her deed would be remembered wherever the Gospel would be preached.

Therapeutic/Medicinal Uses

Spikenard is known to be antibacterial, antifungal, anti-inflammatory, a deodorant, and a skin tonic. It aids in Candida, insomnia, menstrual difficulties, migraines, nausea, rashes, and scar tissues. Spikenard is 93% sesquiterpenes in content, and can erase incorrect information in the DNA or cellular memory.[34]

Dr. Dietrich Gumbel has reported Spikenard being helpful with the heart and circulatory system.[35] It is very relaxing and acts as a natural sedative.

---

[34] <u>Essential Oils Desk Reference</u>. Essential Science Publishing. Page 72.
[35] Dietrich Gumbel, Ph.D.

Aloes/Sandalwood

Aloes is a resin formed as a result of a fungus attack in the heartwood of the Agarwood tree, which takes hundreds of years to develop and is extremely rare and costly.

The meaning of the Arabic word "Aloes" is "little tents." The definition derives from the triangular shape of the capsules from the lingaloes trees. Its resin provides this fragrant spice.

The small tent signified here is a tent on the housetop, a place of intimacy, sometimes called a bridal tent (2 Samuel 16:22, Song of Solomon 4:14). This theme of Aloes referring to the place of intimacy is in Proverbs 7:17: "I have perfumed my bed with myrrh, aloes, and cinnamon."

This fragrance is found in Scripture in John 19:39 after Yeshua's death: "And there came also Nicodemus, which at the first came to Jesus by night, and brought a mixture of myrrh and aloes, about an hundred pound *weight*."

It is interesting to note that 100 pounds of Aloes and Myrrh would be worth $150,000 - $200,000 in today's market. This shows

Nicodemus placed tremendous value and reverence upon the Savior.[36]

Therapeutic/Medicinal Uses

Aloes/Sandalwood is known to support the nerves and circulation and has the ability to stimulate the pineal gland and the limbic region of the brain, the center of emotions. Aloes/Sandalwood can be used for depression and meditation.[37]

This oil can be used for bronchitis, cystitis, skin tumors, urinary tract infection, acne, pulmonary infection, menstrual problems, nervous tension, and skin conditions.[38]

---

[36] "The Life of Jesus Christ" Collectors Edition, Disc 2. Courtesy of Diamond Entertainment, copyrighted.
[37] Ibid.
[38] Essential Oils Desk Reference. Essential Science Publishing. Page 70.

Spice Chest: A Holy Priesthood

The instructions God gave to Moses regarding the fragrances to use for the holy anointing oil are found in Exodus 30:22-31:

"Moreover the LORD spake unto Moses saying, Take thou also unto thee principal spices, of pure myrrh five hundred *shekels*, and of sweet cinnamon half so much, *even* two hundred and fifty *shekels*, and of sweet calamus two hundred and fifty *shekels*, and of cassia five hundred *shekels*, after the shekel of the sanctuary, and of oil olive an hin: and thou shalt make it an oil of holy ointment, an ointment compound after the art of the apothecary: it shall be an holy anointing oil. And thou shalt anoint the tabernacle of the congregation therewith, and the ark of the testimony, and the table and all his vessels, and the candlestick and his vessels, and the altar of incense, and the altar of burnt offering with all his vessels, and the laver and his foot. And thou shalt sanctify them, that they may be most holy: whatsoever toucheth them shall be holy. And thou shalt anoint Aaron and his sons, and consecrate them, that *they* may minister unto me in the priest's office. And thou shalt speak unto the children of Israel, saying, This shall be an holy anointing oil unto me throughout your generations."

During the Mosaic period, special oils were designated by God as the holy anointing oil to sanctify an entire Hebraic genealogy known as the Cohanim priests. The ritual anointing of these priests distinguished them not only for Temple service but, according to Rabbi Aryeh Kaplan, registered in the DNA of their cells which has continued throughout all generations.

In an article entitled "Lost Tribes of Israel," Nova Online reported on the existence of a distinctive Y chromosome in the DNA of Aaron's descendants:

"Genetic studies among Cohanim from all over the world reveal the truth behind this oral tradition. About 50 percent of Cohanim in both Sephardic and Ashkenazic populations have an unusual set of genetic markers on their Y chromosome. What is equally striking is that this genetic signature of the Cohanim is rarely found outside the Jewish populations."

They also stated that rabbis at the Western Wall in Jerusalem took swab tests of Jewish males desiring to know if they are a part of the tribe of Levi in preparation for the third Temple.[39]

---

[39] "Lost Tribes of Israel." Public Broadcasting: Nova Online. http://www.pbs.org/whbh/nova/israelifamilycohanim.html

Cypress

Just as Cedarwood is symbolic of strength, Cypress is also known for strength and durability. These trees were described in the apocryphal book of Siroch as "trees which groweth up to the clouds." The Hebrew word for "Cypress" is *tirzah*, which means "make slender."

The Bible tells that the wood used for Noah's ark was "gopher wood" in Genesis 6:14: "Make thee an ark of gopher wood; rooms shalt thou make in the ark, and shalt pitch it within and without with pitch." It was thought to be Cypress because of its ability to stand up to adverse conditions. Building anything that big would require trees that reached the clouds!

Isaiah 60:13 tells how Cypress represents the sanctuary of the holy feet of God in the coming messianic kingdom: "The glory of Lebanon shall come unto thee, the fir tree, the pine tree, and the box together, to beautify the place of my sanctuary; and I will make the place of my feet glorious."

Therapeutic/Medicinal Uses

The therapeutic qualities of Cypress include improving circulation, supporting the nerves and intestines, and supporting the immune system and cardiovascular system.[40]

Cypress is a good defense against arthritis, bronchitis, cramps, hemorrhoids, insomnia, intestinal parasites, menopausal symptoms, menstrual pain, pancreas insufficiencies, pulmonary infections, throat problems, varicose veins, fluid retention, and scar tissue. It is known to be anti-infectious, antibacterial, and antimicrobial. It strengthens blood capillaries and is good for teeth and gums.

Cypress helps ease the feeling of loss and creates a sense of security. It also brings healing to one during emotional trauma.

---

[40] Essential Oils Desk Reference. Essential Science Publishing. Page 43.

Galbanum

In Exodus 30:34-36 the instructions for the mixing of the holy incense are given:

> "And the LORD said unto Moses, Take unto thee sweet spices, stacte, and onycha, and galbanum; *these* sweet spices with pure frankincense: of each shall there be a like *weight*: and thou shalt make it a perfume, a confection after the art of the apothecary, tempered together, pure *and* holy: and thou shalt beat *some* of it very small, and put of it before the testimony in the tabernacle of the congregation, where I will meet with thee: it shall be unto you most holy."

The Old Testament Apocrypha dating back to BC 180 mentions the formula for holy incense in Sirach 24:15, 1,000 years after Moses.

Most of the spices and perfumes that made up the Temple incense were lovely and fragrant, but Galbanum had a more earthy, parsley-like smell. The Jewish Talmud suggests that Galbanum—a less than wonderful fragrant resin—was included in the holy incense because "every communal fast that does not include the sinners of Israel is not a fast."

The Hebrew word for "Galbanum" is *cheleb*, which means "the fat or the richest part." The Torah instructed the priest that when he offered up the goat as an offering made by fire for a sweet aroma, all the *cheleb* (the fat) belonged to the Lord and was forbidden for human consumption.

Believers are to be "lean" and to avoid fulfilling their lusts of worldly affections. The excess Yah gives a believer is to be offered back up to Him to complete His mission and ministry on the earth, not for believers to be lazy and gluttonous with.

Therapeutic/Medicinal Uses

The essential oil of Galbanum is anti-infectious, anti-inflammatory, and analgesic.[41] It supports the kidneys and a woman's menstrual cycle. It is also helpful with asthma, poor circulation, wounds, acne, bronchitis, cramps, indigestion, muscular aches and pains, nervous tension, scar tissue, and wrinkles.

Galbanum has been reported to bring harmony and balance, easing stress. It helps increase spiritual awareness and meditation.

---

[41] Essential Oils Desk Reference. Essential Science Publishing. Page 49.

Spice Chest: Duties of the Cohanim

The Scriptures tell that the original healers/physicians of the Bible were the priests, who often anointed the sick and prayed for them. The role of the priesthood where they diagnosed, prescribed, and administered oils is described in Leviticus 13 and 14.

Their duties included: leading worship, receiving tithes, making sacrifices, and offering up prayers on behalf of the saints as spiritual counselors and hearers of confession. The Levites were to keep the fire burning day and night, taking care of the Temple of God. They mixed various oils for incense, healing, and anointing, and offered medicinal diagnosis and treatment. Their life was to exemplify righteousness.

The duties described for the priests in Leviticus and 1 Chronicles 9:26-30 actually describe the same responsibilities given to the Bride of Messiah, who is a priest as well.

1 Peter 2:9 says, "But ye *are* a chosen generation, a royal priesthood, an holy nation." And in Revelation 1:6 says, "And hath made us kings and priests unto God and his Father; to him *be* glory and dominion for ever and ever. Amen."

As priests, followers of Yeshua must keep the fire in their hearts burning passionately for Him and are instructed to pray for and anoint the sick, just as the Cohanim did.

The Bible says in 1 Corinthians 3:16 it says, "Know ye not that ye are the temple of God, and *that* the Spirit of God dwelleth in you?" The body of a believer is the Temple of the Holy Spirit, and the believer is to keep his Temple—the body—attractive and in good repair. As a holy instrument, believers can anoint themselves to be sanctified vessels for God's use.

Frankincense

Pure and holy biblical incense contains genuine Frankincense, which burns with ascending white smoke. Revelation 8:3-4 says that the original altar of incense continues to be used before the throne of God in Heaven.

Frankincense represents the godly prayers of His people rising to the throne (Exodus 30:1-9; Revelation 5:8). As ministers of the Lord, the priests burned incense before the ark in the Holy of Holies.

The Hebrew word *lebonah* means "incense," which is Frankincense. There are five other places in the Bible where *lebonah* was translated "incense," meaning Frankincense. The Hebrew word for "Frankincense" means "pure or white." This is because of the milk-colored drops of aromatic resin that flow from the slashed inner wood of the tree.

The Boswellia Olibanum tree, which produces Frankincense, takes forty years to mature. In July 2006, the Tampa Tribune reported an over-harvesting of the trees and how the next generation isn't producing seedlings. The book of Revelation says that these oils will cease in the last days.

Pure Frankincense was also placed on the loaves of bread to symbolize the purity and fragrance of Christ, the true Bread of God (Leviticus 24:5-7, John 6:32-33, Exodus 30:34-36). A portion of this prescribed incense was not burned but simply placed before the ark in the Holy of Holies. God said that this is "where I shall meet with you; it shall be holy (the holiest) to you." This represented the prayers in Heaven between Yeshua God's Son and the Heavenly Father.

In Numbers 16:46-50, it reads:

"And Moses said unto Aaron, Take a censer, and put fire therein from off the altar, and put on incense, and go quickly unto the congregation, and make an atonement for them: for there is wrath gone out from the LORD; the plague is begun. And Aaron took as Moses commanded, and ran into the midst of the congregation; and, behold, the plague was begun among the people: and he put on incense, and made an atonement for the people. And he stood between the dead and the living; and the plague was stayed. Now they that died in the plague were fourteen thousand and seven hundred, beside them that died about the matter of Korah. And Aaron returned unto Moses unto the door of the tabernacle of the congregation: and the plague was stayed."

This incense used by Aaron in the book of Numbers stopped the plague from spreading. Believers can follow this example to protect themselves from the coming plagues in the last days.

The Gift of Frankincense

Frankincense was not only used for incense, but was offered as a gift. In Isaiah 60:3, Isaiah prophesied of the Magi's gifts: "And the Gentiles shall come to thy light, and kings to the brightness of thy rising." And verse 6 continues, "The multitude of camels shall cover thee, the dromedaries of Midian and Ephah; all they from Sheba shall come: they shall bring gold and incense; and they shall shew forth the praises of the LORD."

The Magi's arrival is seen in Matthew 2:11:

"And when they were come into the house, they saw the young child with Mary his mother, and fell down, and worshipped him: and when they had opened their treasures, they presented unto him gifts; gold, and frankincense, and myrrh."

Mary and Joseph may have used the gifts to help protect Yeshua, keeping Him strong and healthy.

A Pure Cure-all

The Egyptians considered Frankincense to be a universal cure-all, used for everything from gout to a broken head—in other words, from "head to toe."

In northern Egypt, a sect of Jews called "Theraputei" continue to practice the healing arts by anointing the sick with oils and laying hands on them, as Yeshua did in His adult life.

Therapeutic/Medicinal Uses

Fumigation was one of the ways biblical people used essential oils—today, diffusers create the same effect.

Frankincense is safe to inhale, rub on the skin, and to take internally. It supports the immune system.[42] The Arabs make teeth-whitening chewing gum from this resin. Frankincense heals cuts and wounds and also cures the common cold.

Today, Frankincense is used in many perfumes and colognes including the best-selling men's fragrance "Old Spice" and Estee Lauder's "Youth Dew."

Uses for this oil include asthma, headaches, hemorrhaging, high blood pressure, tonsillitis, warts, allergies, cancer, ulcers, bronchitis, and respiratory infections.

Frankincense essential oils stimulate and elevate the mind. It overcomes stress and despair.[43]

---

[42] Essential Oils Desk Reference. Essential Science Publishing. Page 48.
[43] Ibid.

Spice Chest: Anointing that Breaks the Yoke

Psalm 133:2 it describes the anointing of Aaron with "precious ointment upon the head, that ran down upon the beard, *even* Aaron's beard: that went down to the skirts of his garments." The words "precious" and "ointment" indicate that this was not just olive oil but pure oils such as were used in the holy anointing oil.[44]

The Hebrew word for "anoint" is *masach*, which means "to smear, spread, or massage," and in some cases it means "to pour oil over the head or body." It shares the same root term as "Messiah," *mashiyach*, meaning "anointed one." In the New Testament, the Greek word *kristos* or "Christ" means "anointed one" and is used 361 times.

Other words and phrases used in the Scriptures such as anointing oil, ointment, spices, incense, perfumes, odors or sweet savors, aromas, or fragrances, all imply essential oils.

A unique act of anointing is found in ancient Chinese medicine—for thousands of years they have placed oil on the inside of the ear and this place was called the "sheman" point. Yahweh instructed anointing this point of the right ear in Leviticus 14:17:

---

[44] "The Old Testament: Volume Four." A David Solomon and Elijah Vanguard video, copyright 1997.

"And the rest of the oil that *is* in his hand shall the priest put upon the tip of the right ear of him that is to be cleansed, and upon the thumb of his right hand, and upon the great toe of his right foot, upon the blood of the trespass offering."

This practice was used in a cleansing ceremony for leprosy to cleanse the leper and his house, and in another ceremony to release emotional patterns of guilt. Both of these rituals involved Cedarwood, Hyssop, and a "log of oil" (10 fluid ounces) which would have been beaten olive oil containing aromatics. Modern research has found that this portion of the ear is where one releases and resolves issues of guilt regarding their parents.

The biblical act of anointing is mentioned 156 times in the Bible. The Hebrew word for "anointing" is *shemen*, which means "fat oil, fatness, or olive oil." In Isaiah 10:27, it says, "And it shall come to pass in that day, *that* his burden shall be taken away from off thy shoulder, and his yoke from off they neck, and the yoke shall be destroyed because of the anointing." It is the *oil* that breaks the yoke.

Myrtle

Esther 2:7 says:

"And he brought up Hadassah, that *is*, Esther, his uncle's daughter: for she had neither father nor mother, and the maid *was* fair and beautiful; whom Mordecai, when her father and mother were dead, took for his own daughter."

The Hebrew word *Hadassah*, Esther's Hebrew name, means "Myrtle." Because the Bible mentions this, she probably used Myrtle during her preparation for its therapeutic qualities of balancing the hormones.

Myrtle is also a treasured herb used in the celebration of the Feast of Tabernacles (the Feast of *Sukkot* mentioned in Nehemiah 8:15 and Zechariah 14:16).

Myrtle is a picture of *Elohim Echad*, as seen in Deuteronomy 6:4, "Hear, O Israel: The LORD our God *is* one LORD." Its leaves are in clusters of groups of threes, but all grow from the same point on the stem. The Hebrew word *echad* means "one comprised of more than one." The leaves of the Myrtle plant are a picture of the Father, Son and *Ruach HaKodesh*—the Holy Spirit—as it says in Deuteronomy 6:4.

Therapeutic/Medicinal Uses

The oil of Myrtle is effective for normalizing hormonal imbalances of the thyroid, hypothyroid, and ovaries, as well as soothing the respiratory system.[45] The therapeutic properties of Myrtle show that it is anti-infectious, a liver stimulant, eases prostate, is a decongestant, and a skin tonic.[46]

Myrtle has been used to help with asthma, sinus and respiratory infections, tuberculosis, hormone imbalances, and hypothyroidism.

Myrtle is very helpful for clearing anger.

---

[45] Essential Oils Desk Reference. Essential Science Publishing. Page 61.
[46] Ibid.

Onycha

Onycha comes from the Balsam or Benzoin Tree of the Far East. However, rabbis debate whether Onycha is a resin from a tree. Some believe it is an aromatic from a mussel or shell because of its Hebraic root. Others, such as Rabbi Gamaliel (whom the Apostle Paul studied under), believe it is actually a part of the balsam species.

The Hebrew word "Onycha" is *shecheleth*, which means "part of the holy incense, sweet kind of gum, and shines as the nail." Because of this definition, some believe Onycha comes from the same mussel which provides the purplish-blue color used to dye tzitzits or fringes on the prayer shawl.

As seen in Exodus 30:34, Onycha is used in the holy anointing oil. It is also mentioned in the Talmud and the Old Testament Apocrypha.

According to Strong's Concordance, it is from the same root word as *shachal*, meaning "to roar; a lion from its characteristic roar." This describes Yeshua, the Lion of the tribe of Judah! The Lord has been given all authority in Heaven and Earth as the Lion of Judah (Matthew 28:18 and Revelation 5:5).

Onycha is one of the heaviest oils and is too thick to pour. Its scent will seem familiar to some because it contains vanillin aldehyde, which gives it a vanilla scent.

Therapeutic/Medicinal Uses

Healing properties of Onycha include: anti-inflammatory, antioxidant, and antiseptic. It combats arthritis, gout, asthma, bronchitis, and skin conditions.[47]

The author of Aromatherapy Solutions writes that Onycha was used for thousands of years for respiratory conditions.[48] Many have used it for poor circulation, flu, chills, colic, coughs, and skin conditions such as chapped or inflamed skin.

Onycha is valued for its ability to speed the healing of wounds and prevent infection. Other names it is called include: "Friar's Balm," "Benzoin," and "Java Frankincense."[49]

The fragrance of Onycha is a reminder to Satan that he is a defeated foe and believers share in the Lord's authority "to tread on... all the power of the enemy" in His name (Luke 10:19).

---

[47] Stewart, David, Ph.D., D.N.M. Healing Oils of the Bible. Care Publications. 2003.
[48] Aromatherapy Solutions.
[49] Essential Oils Desk Reference. Essential Science Publishing.

Spice Chest: Virgin Olive Oil

Olive oil is used as a carrier oil and the Bible clearly states that the only grade of olive oil suitable for holy anointing purposes is the "first oil." The Bible discusses this in Leviticus 24:2: "Command the children of Israel, that they bring unto thee pure oil olive beaten for the light, to cause the lamps to burn continually."

Today, first oil is called "virgin oil." Virgin olive oil has a wonderful fragrance and flavor. First oil is not pressed from the fruit but drained from the crushed fruit.

The "first oil" or virgin oil serves as a spiritual picture of the Bride of Messiah. She is the first to come out of Babylon on her own and is drawn by the *Ruach*. The Bride has a fragrance the world recognizes as different.

The second oil, or "pressed oil," is inferior and its fruit is crushed, stamped, and squeezed to get the very last drop of oil. This oil was not acceptable as an offering to the Temple—as it has no flavor or fragrance.

Believers who are sluggish and foolish have to be beaten and endure fiery trials like the second oil to come out.

The choice still remains theirs. Will a believer be a fragrant offering to Him or be hard-pressed and remain tasteless to the world? 2 Corinthians 2:14-15 says, "Now thanks *be* unto God, which always causeth us to triumph in Christ, and maketh manifest the savour of his knowledge by us in every place. For we are unto God a sweet savour of Christ."

Index

CPSIA information can be obtained at www.ICGtesting.com
Printed in the USA
BVOW06s0933250715

410134BV00007B/95/P